The
HRT for
MEN
Imperatives

The HRT for MEN Imperatives

"A must-read for every man over 55, and for the women and men who love them"

by Glynn Christian

Why 55+ Men's Health Needs Testosterone-Replacement Therapy

Written with the first-hand authority of a man who was once robbed of his testosterone and became a Testosterone-Pauper

ISBN 9781795874274

Dedication

This book is dedicated to the relief of the unjustified suffering
of the Silent Horde of countless hundreds of thousands
of living men who suffer Testosterone-Poverty
and to the memory of the unimaginable numbers of those
who painfully preceded them.

Contents

PART ONE

A Silent Horde of Testosterone-Pauper Tragedies

Oblivion of Knowledge

There is a Silent Horde of men world-wide, men who are suffering unheard because their symptoms of low-testosterone levels are unrecognised and untreated. These might include depression, osteoporosis, loss of numeracy or spatial skills and many others. Yes, these do include erectile dysfunction or lack of libido, too, but surprisingly these are not often the major complaints of sufferers.

It's an avoidable situation but much of the world's medical profession seem not to be aware that these men's symptoms are associated with low-testosterone levels or knowledgeable about what they might do to alleviate them.

Members of that Silent Horde are not the men they should be and could be. They're castrates or near castrates and the implications are dire. They are Testosterone-Paupers. Despair, heartbreak and potential suicide are implicit.

An endemic oblivion in men's health knowledge results in countless Testosterone-Pauper Tragedies, heartbreak in every country of the world.

A Man Doesn't Need to Lose His Balls

First, let's be clear that a man doesn't have to lose his balls to be a complete Testosterone-Pauper, the modern man's equivalent of history's eunuch. I was impoverished by having my testosterone removed chemically, rather than being tangibly castrated, as preparation for prostate-cancer treatment. I was not properly warned of the possible physical and mental consequences.

They were awful and some are lifelong.

At the bottom of my despair I realised that every year there are hundreds of thousands of other men worldwide, millions probably, who are undergoing treatment for prostate cancer and who have been so treated. Many were likely to be suffering some or all of my horrid symptoms, the rupture of my personal and business lives, and an absolute erasure of my self-worth and of my identity.

Where Were Their Voices? Was Anyone Listening? Who Cared?

Answers from within the medical fraternity were equivocal. Most prevaricated or obstructed – anything to avoid the truth it now seems. In my view this was sometimes to protect their income, other times to disguise lack of knowledge about testosterone and the possible effects of its sudden erasure.

Then, I discovered incalculably many more men were suffering the Living Hell of Age-related Testosterone-Poverty, all of them sentenced simply because they have grown older than men had ever done before.

Thus, it is imperative to unbox medicine's greatest modern secret, that there are more eunuchs or Testosterone-Paupers living in the 21st century than at any time in history, just as undiscovered and just as pained as history's millions of physical eunuchs. That's simply because there are more old men alive today than at any time in history.

Getting the Facts Clear and Why Families and Friends Matter, too

A Testosterone-Pauper is a man of any age, whose testicles have slowed or stopped the production of testosterone, the male hormone that first designs and then fuels everything to do with his masculinity.

Genetically, every man is born different and will manufacture more or less testosterone. This is not proportionate to his body size, his penis size or the size and weight of his testicles. Equally unequal, men begin to lose about 1% - some sources say more - of their testosterone from around the age of 30. This natural attrition rarely deletes a man's testosterone completely but the loss is relentless, inescapable.

Without active testicles a man's body loses far more than sperm factories and reproductive ability. His testosterone is reduced or lost and thus he cannot be the man he was meant to be. When he totally stops producing testosterone, this is known as Primary Hypo-gonadism.

Testosterone-Paupers have less or very little of the driving force of testosterone, the widely misunderstood or ignored state I call Testosterone-Poverty. In extreme cases Testosterone-Poverty is absolute. Victims are the equivalent of physical castrates and may as well not have testicles, like the equally silent, adult-made eunuchs of history, whose voices are now barely distant whispers but that were once infuriated roars. Grumpy old men are not being difficult on purpose; they simply might not have enough testosterone to keep them happy. Does your GP know this?

What Testosterone-Replacement Therapy Can Do

If a man develops prostate cancer, testosterone is widely considered unkindly to feed the tumour, plumping it with encouragement so it rudely bursts from the prostate and conquers all it encounters and thus kills. The research supporting the connection between prostate cancer and testosterone is very old and modern forensic techniques would be likely to redefine this, suggesting alternative targeted treatments rather than the single blunt instrument of immediate testosterone suppression after diagnosis but before treatment.

Apart from the direct physical and mental effects of Testosterone-Poverty, an ageing man can suffer great torment. Inevitable changes to his personal relationships, sporting prowess or business life, combined with a dearth of diagnostic understanding or compassion plus little or no treatment, can enrage him, so he becomes angry, aggressive and difficult to live with.

Thus, the families, friends and work colleagues of Testosterone-Paupers suffer, too. The discomforts of this wider circle should equally be ameliorated and are prime reasons for wider understanding of Testosterone-Poverty and the advantages of HRT for MEN, the maintenance of testosterone levels.

It's time Testosterone-Paupers and those around them spoke up, are spoken up for, are listened to, and then helped to become productive, sociable, capable and caring men again.

Testosterone-Replacement Therapy would do that, would restore vitality and self-worth in many of the ways a man has lost, from once again driving safely to restored numerical and spatial ability, yes and erectile function, too, if that is what he wants.

PART TWO

The Proper Role of Testosterone

Slithery Spectrums

Testosterone is a brute, the malicious, masterless master of every man. Provided he has some.

Fully to understand what it's like to be a man or to be a Testosterone-Pauper in any degree, you must appreciate the role of testosterone, one of the male body's main androgens or sex hormones. Understanding testosterone means you should never be outwitted by the ignorance or obstruction of others.

As an adult male, 95% of testosterone production is controlled by the pea-sized pituitary gland which sits at the base of the brain and commands the testicles to manufacture and dispense the hormone, explaining why men with cancer or disorders of that organ can experience degrees of Testosterone-Poverty without anything being wrong with their testicles.

Testosterone is also made by the small, potent adrenal glands that sit on top of the kidneys but the amount these might contribute – about 5% - is not enough to continue erectile virility after castration, whether physical, chemical or accidental, except in the very rarest of cases and then not for long.

From the split-second strike of conception, all foetuses are inherently female, the default of the human race, and thus all have nipples. Each is quickly about the size of a raindrop, with a heart beating 150 times a minute, but difference is deeply embedded.

Some foetuses have XX chromosomes and are meant to become female; some have XY chromosomes and are predicated to be male. Around an eight-12 week point, the inherited imperatives of the mother's genome configuration mean an XY embryo gets a shot of testosterone from her that tells it to develop a penis and testicles rather than a clitoris and ovaries; the foetus is disposed to develop into a male, more or less.

That first tiny, bullying dose of testosterone in the womb initiates hard wiring of the differences between male and female brains and decrees absolutely the future rites of passage that mean, during the puberty of the boy-child, his maturing testicles distribute new supplies of testosterone to ensure his proto-man's shoulders should widen and hips stay narrow. His face should become bearded and his throat should swell to create an Adam's apple and deeper voice.

Continuous testosterone from his dropped and burgeoning testicles should then enhance his brain's predestined capacity for such largely male-centric skills as numeracy and science-oriented cognitive and spatial abilities, of driving and map reading, of imagining and designing buildings or furniture or space rockets.

I say that's what should happen but the infinite variability of human DNA inherited by the XY foetus, plus the greater or lesser amount of testosterone received so early, will ultimately produce a male human who has a unique place somewhere on the slithery spectrums of gender and sexuality.

Nature, Nuture or Nastiness

If the mother provided too little testosterone, the foetus is only part-masculinised and will grow up to be equivocal, physically, mentally or sexually.

None of us had a choice. There is no absolute in this lottery and it also seems the odds can be changed by outside influence.

For countless centuries, competitive women in Ottoman harems believed frightening a pregnant woman during the early months of gestation interfered with the natural development of the unborn baby. Aeons of observation had persuaded them that, if the damaged foetus turned out to be a boy, it would then grow up feminised or homosexual and thus be less likely to want, or be allowed, to win the throne; inheritance by the oldest son was by no means assured, even if he was lucky enough still to be living.

From Topkapi's sea-breeze-swept pavilions to the oppressive single-storey palaces of Beijing's Forbidden City, the sovereign's mother often had as much or more power then her regnant son. There are cases of Chinese empresses deliberately encouraging eunuchs to further weaken a sickly heir or actual emperor with drugs and debauchery, so their own powers were less trammelled.

The received knowledge of Topkapi's persecuting women may

have been right. It seems fright really can reduce the amount of testosterone a mother feeds her *in utero* foetus. After the Second World War, research was done on German women who had felt threatened and fearful during Berlin air raids while in early pregnancy, and it found a higher percentage of their sons was homosexual than the norm. (The Guardian: August 29th 2005).

The combined effects of testosterone and genetic inheritance on foetal development are so capricious that some children appear totally female in every physical aspect until they are about 12, when what seem to be labial folds and a clitoris disappear and working testicles and a penis appear; the *guevadoces* (eggs at 12) of the Dominican Republic are the best known examples.

So, testosterone, or a lack of it, is responsible for most differences between men and women and affects conditions far more varied and variable than most of us ever imagined, from osteoporosis to mental health. And yes, testosterone levels given in the womb do explain why many women are quite as good as men at many technical, mathematical and other spatial-based skills.

These intrinsic birth differences explain why every man will experience different symptoms from any attrition of his testosterone levels. A man who has always had low levels of testosterone might well seem largely unaffected as he grows older or is treated for prostate cancer.

Differing natural testosterone levels explain the huge diversity there is in the apparent masculinity or femininity seen in men but that have nothing to do with their sexual orientation. The arching range of adult-male appearance, manner and sexual preference is largely directed by the testosterone balance given them early in the womb, indeed Nature rather than nurture.

This explains why some men have piping, girly voices, even though very masculine looking. Their testosterone simply did not get around to widening their voice boxes and thus deepening their voices. It is probably a factor in the unsettling voice quality of many effeminate and possibly homosexual men.

Angry Eunuchs

Of the many awful mental and physical side effects of castration and thus of complete Testosterone-Poverty, men will have little or no sex drive, be incapable of erections. Such sexual impotence is not the sole explanation for the generally hateful dismissal of history's Invisible Horde of Eunuchs as bad-tempered, avaricious and cruel, but no book I know has looked deeper, no writer has bothered to ask why eunuchs so often behaved badly. They never troubled to discover that eunuchs' behaviour was and is a direct result of Testosterone-Poverty and its side effects, as outlined later in this book in A Catechism of Testosterone-Poverty. As more 21st-century men live longer than any other men in history, natural erosion of testosterone is silently disintegrating the thin veil between modern men with testicles and history's eunuchs, ex- males with none.

Further to Fall

Eunuchs are rarely spoken of these days. Most people today know nothing of the suffering they endured. A greater proportion had been castrated before they were ten years old, and the effects of this are quite different from adult-made castrates. Testosterone controls aspects of pubertal bone growth and when it should stop. Throughout history, when average heights were far less, a pre-pubertal eunuch could grow to well over six feet (1.8288 metres) as well as suffering weak muscle development and almost certain osteoporosis. These weaknesses made them more likely to fall and then gave them far further to fall.

In the West we know mainly of the sensational voices and careers of those few castrati who became superstars, dominating European stages, including those of London during the Baroque 17th and 18th centuries. Farinelli and Seresino were just two; the latter was regularly mocked in contemporary prints for extreme height, his humped back, barrel chest and his long legs with knock-knees that were simply too weak properly to support his bulk.

I am regularly astonished at how little Registrars/junior doctors know about testosterone, even in specialist endocrinology clinics; one even asked me how castration could have affected the singing voices of the famed castrati stars.

In case you don't know, the body of a boy castrated between the ages of eight and ten or so ages without further testosterone and thus does not go through puberty. His throat does not develop the normal way with an Adam's apple and his voice does not break.

The bones of his chest, like his legs and arms, over-develop and then adult-sized lungs propel a great amount of air through his boy's throat. With intense training his unnaturally powerful and high boy's singing voice could be so beautiful, so flexible and so sustainable that castrati opera stars were commonly greeted with the cry 'Long live the knife'.

It's said that women fainted and men swooned when such as Farinelli held a soprano note for over a minute while also creating spontaneous embellishments and variations. Castrati voices seemed supernatural, some would say angelic, which explains their long popularity within the choirs of the Catholic Church in Italy, especially that of the Vatican's Sistine Chapel.

Oddly, these maimed curiosities, who had never been men and who had sensational high and pure voices, were cast on operatic stages throughout Europe as such great male heroes as Julius Caesar and Alexander the Great. Baroque sensibilities somehow equated their supernatural voices with the extraordinary achievements of these supermen-conquerors.

Singers who had been castrated as children were a common part of court, religious and urban British and European life in the 17th and 18th centuries and not just as performers. The Italian castrato star Tenducci became director of the Handel festivals at Westminster Abbey for King George III. He actually married, a 15-year old Irish girl called Dorothea Maunsell. She subsequently obtained a divorce, very rare for the times, on the grounds of non-consummation, famously describing his penis as looking like a 'small white worm'.

That fact alone should be enough (but isn't) to stamp out the silliness of thinking castrati made fabulous but sterile lovers. To sing like they did, they had to have been castrated before puberty and thus would never have grown anything with which to penetrate man or woman. Neither would they have had the hormones that stimulated libido or erectile flesh.

For centuries, the uncanny yet angelic voices of pre-pubertal eunuchs were vital to the Catholic Church, which forbade women in their choirs. Only in 1878 did Pope Leo XIII outlaw the hiring of new castrati to sing in the Sistine Chapel of the Vatican but it was almost 25 years more, in 1902, before the church stopped using the castrati who were already employed.

Emperors Dominated

The labyrinthine palaces of the Ottoman and the Chinese Empires employed eunuchs well into the 20th century. Often these had been castrated when young adults, a choice commonly given to criminals in China instead of them losing a hand or their lives. They lived, but who today has ever thought of what they suffered because of sudden Testosterone-Poverty when castrated at what's considered the height of virility? Who has matched Testosterone-Poverty to their often hideous bad-temper and brutality? Just imagine how ill-temper and envy caused through testosterone loss and the complete obliteration of their masculinity affected the history of the empires they supposedly served.

It was always eunuchs who were closest to any emperor, to his young sons, his empresses and his countless concubines, because no whole man could sleep in such as Beijing's Forbidden City. The eunuchs had many unsupervised, candle-lit hours to scheme and plot, to whisper into opium-fumed ears, to create drug addictions and disaffection and favourites. And to amass huge personal fortunes.

The 16th century eunuch Liu Jin so dominated his young emperor Wu-Tsung that he was once able to express his spite by beheading 300 bureaucrats who didn't agree to his wish for a eunuch-dominated political hierarchy. Liu amassed such an immense private fortune, including several solid-gold suits of armour, that when discovered and assessed its overall value equated to the same amount as Imperial China's annual budget.

Adult-made eunuchs were often defeated soldiers or captured citizens and thus they would suffer the severest effects outlined in The Catechism of Testosterone-Poverty Symptoms. To these must be added their unimaginable mental sufferings, including anger and desire for revenge for their emasculation as adults, and the emotional pain of separation from home and families, of enslavement and then of base servitude.

The extraordinary and quite unsuspected saga of history's Invisible Horde of eunuchs is my next book: CUT! *The Pained Life and Loves of History's Eunuchs.*

The essential point of historic human castration was to make males incapable of fathering a child. A modern vasectomy, the severing of the vas deferens, means men will no longer include sperm in their ejaculations yet will retain their ability to manufacture testosterone, thus avoiding any of the mental and physical side effects of losing all testicular functions. In every purpose other than procreation, they are still whole men. They can still get prostate cancer.

Historic castration was not focussed. It was blunt and blind, everything or nothing. What worked with animals was supposed to work with men. It's not as simple as that because human testosterone is utterly unsympathetic. However you lose it, you will be punished, even if the loss is supposedly saving your life.

The Duchess Question

Even when it is present, testosterone can play games.

Some male (XY) foetuses have an insensitivity (allergy would be the modern but incorrect word) to the transformative power of testosterone and so their expected masculine characteristics do not develop fully and much of the foetus's default female state remains.

Vanity Fair magazine published an article proposing this as an explanation for why the American Wallis Warfield, later Duchess of Windsor, appeared both masculine and feminine, a possibility also raised in several biographies of this fascinating wife of ex-King Edward VIII of Great Britain, created HRH the Duke of Windsor after he relinquished the throne for love of Wallis.

The magazine said post-mortem x-rays of the duchess's skeleton proved she should have been a man but that a degree of androgen insensitivity must have prevented male sexual organs developing.

Instead, they said, her inherent female sexual organs developed but not enough so that she could menstruate or conceive.

They also wrote that children who played with Wallis Warfield in her Baltimore hometown said that she had a knot of tissue where they had proper boy and girl bits to toy with and to compare.

As a young woman Wallis went to China and was there rumoured to have learned advanced sexual technique, particularly that of fellatio, said to be an uncommon interest of Western women at the time. Or was it some physical anomaly that she had sorted out in China?

Earl Mountbatten, whispered to have enough first-hand knowledge of male genitalia to make reliable comparisons, once said that the duchess's husband had the smallest 'willy' he'd ever seen.

So, was it shared physical inadequacies that gratefully stuck the Duke and Duchess of Windsor together?

It is one of the many mysteries about the fascinating duchess that none of her three husbands or other rumoured lovers revealed the truth. Neither did any of the married women who had previously shared Edward's bed ever tell tales. Or perhaps neither of her husbands, nor his or her reputed lovers, nor their many servants, ever gossiped because there were never stories to be told and that Edward and Wallis were simply a man and a woman truly in love.

Drag-Queens, Fingers and Twins

Low-testosterone levels possibly explain why you rarely see a short drag-queen. Have you noticed, even before the outrageous heels and wigs, these are almost always tall but feminised men, often with a characteristic quacky or reedy voice? Their height and voice could both be a symptom of their bodies always having had low testosterone levels.

Testosterone plays an important part in determining height. Without a determined full-stop by the hormone during puberty, gristle pads at the end of long bones continue to turn into bone for much longer than they should.

So, big surprise, male height is not always a sign of masculinity but can be a marker of feminisation caused by lack of appropriate levels of testosterone. Equally, low testosterone levels can prevent a boy's throat and voice developing its expected manly potential, leaving him with something permanently 'unbroken' throughout his adulthood.

Then there is the curious question of finger length. It seems that the basic male hand should have an index finger shorter than the ring finger, whereas a woman will generally have a longer index finger than her ring finger.

Thus it might be judged that a man with an index finger longer than his ring finger is likely to be feminised to a greater degree than 'normal' but in what way is impossible to tell by mere observation.

A longer index finger is absolutely not a sign a man is gay, just as a shorter one does not mean a woman is a lesbian, but looking at finger lengths certainly makes hand-watching a fascinating way to pass time, privately or publically.

Sometimes hormones leak between foetuses and that's considered a reason why twin boys, who should be identical, can be uneven heights and sizes, because one has garnered more testosterone. It's more common than usually admitted that one identical boy twin is likely to be homosexual or, at least, to be more susceptible to the charms of his own sex than is his brother, almost certainly influenced by an uneven share of the testosterone received from their mother; this is equally true of fraternal boy twins. Sometimes, a mother gives twin XY foetuses so little testosterone that both boys grow up as homosexual, just as two or more brothers can be gay.

We must all accept that each man's testosterone level is as unpredictable as the throw of dice.

American Journal of Medicine 'behoves'

My Catechism of Testosterone-Poverty itemises the frightening challenges of testosterone loss that might be faced, yet only hints at the poisonous cocktail that can visit. It is based on the findings published in the American Journal of Medicine (2002), given to me by a consultant Harley Street andrologist, who confirmed my many afflictions were based on Testosterone-Poverty, but there are many other sources of reference, easily sourced on the internet.

The most common state is the Age-related Testosterone-Pauper and there are five more categories. All six types of Testosterone-Paupers can be helped with careful, supervised testosterone supplements, HRT for MEN, but this seems feared or, worse, is unrecognised by much of the world's medical profession. High alcohol intake can also contribute to low levels of testosterone, indeed it might be said that Alcohol-related Testosterone-Paupers should be added to the above as a further individual category but alcohol is more often only an additional causative.

The American Journal of Medicine firmly said in 2002 that it 'behoves' the medical profession in every country in the world to get up to date with increasing understanding of testosterone attrition in ageing men and to restore Testosterone-Paupers to fuller independence and back to their social, business and family status.

This is especially true in the careful use of Testosterone-Replacement Therapy as a treatment for 55+ male depression, which is increasingly proven to be linked to Testosterone-Poverty. Without daily Testosterone-Replacement Therapy I would be wrecked, or dead, perhaps by my own hand, which would many times have been a welcome liberation. I am not alone in feeling like that.

That man with undiagnosed Testosterone-Poverty could be any man or woman's grandfather, father or brother, son, grandson or nephew, could be a husband/partner, a work colleague, a lover or a neighbour. Or each of them.

He could even be you.

The tragedies of avoidable Testosterone-Poverty must be told boldly, man to man. We must heed the unheeded cries of today's Silent-Horde, even if only of those we know, and then cry loudly on their behalf. Unfortunately, most men are lamentably lame about admitting weaknesses to themselves or asking for help to solve problems and pains in their bodies. To achieve the greatest support for HRT for MEN, we must acknowledge that women care more for men's health than men do.

Why Women Must Lead the Way

It is paramount that women should listen and look harder for symptoms of Testosterone-Poverty amongst the men in their lives if this silent, world-wide agony is to be recognised and treated with compassion and the recuperative potential of modern medicine.

Together women and men everywhere must battle medical ignorance and demand Testosterone-Replacement Therapy, claiming it as a right, as much a right as HRT is for women. This time, where women once led, men must now follow and do it equally loudly.

So, first let me show you the many ways that Testosterone-Poverty can affect men, my Catechism of Testosterone-Poverty. Then, we'll look at the six quite different ways a man might become a Testosterone-Pauper.

PART THREE

A Catechism
of
Testosterone-Poverty

22 Common Symptoms

All, some or none of the following 22 symptoms of Testosterone-Poverty might occur and each might manifest in minor to major dynamics. This sounds as though diagnosis is difficult but a simple blood test quickly shows up a low-testosterone level. This simple procedure makes it hard to understand why the remedy of Testosterone-Replacement Therapy, HRT for MEN, is so little prescribed, even in medically advanced countries.

On the following pages are some of the symptoms for which you should look. The first two, of altered mood and depression, are probably the most common and most easily identifiable by others. The second two, libido and erectile dysfunction, might well be kept private but are usually partnered by mood change or depression to some degree. If they are minor, symptoms like body-hair loss, weight redistribution or such as changed card-playing skills are not serious hindrances to Quality of Life to many men and are can be accepted as inevitable signs of ageing, as indeed they are.

The symptoms preceded by **!** are the symptoms I suffered, most of them severely, mainly because I was relatively young when my prostate-cancer was diagnosed and thus still had quite high testosterone levels before they were vanquished suddenly. Not every man will have the same experiences, naturally or as a result of prostate-cancer treatment.

A Catechism of Testosterone-Poverty

! Mood swings, including heightened emotional sensitivity manifesting as tearfulness, over-reaction to minor issues and unjustified anger

! Depression in all degrees, from minor grumpiness to major shutdown

! Lowering or loss of libido

! Lowering or loss of erectile ability

! Lightening of voice

! Hot flushes/flashes when testosterone is removed suddenly, as with trauma, disease or with prostate-cancer therapy; these might or might not continue

! Severe sweating episodes by day or night when testosterone is removed suddenly, as with trauma, disease or with prostate-cancer therapy; these usually continue as long as the hot flushes/flashes

! Diminishment of cognitive abilities, including short-term memory, which can contribute to confusion and speech difficulties, including problems in communicating with health professionals; inability to cook threatening health; lack of interest in personal care and living conditions further reduce social interactions and possibility of support

! Numeracy loss including inability to calculate, to count or even to assess money in the hand; business life, card games and simply shopping for food become frightening challenges

! Reduction of spatial (space and distance) sentience, which can mean a reduced ability to draw or design or to understand technical instructions including recipes; loss of orientation skills mean not driving or parking safely; failure to understand maps; easily becoming lost even when walking; diminished capacity to play golf and other sports where calculation of distance is important

! Increased heart rate

Loss of bone mass and potential osteoporosis, which can be accompanied by pain and skeletal disfigurement

! Loss of muscle tone and strength

! Softening and reduction of beard but possible strengthening of head hair

! Loss or softening of body hair except for pubic hair; male-pattern baldness is unlikely to revert

! Skin softening

! Change of fat deposits into female patterns, particularly to the hips

Breast growth, in some cases extreme

Prostate withering

Urinary incontinence, if penis removed by surgery or trauma; ! also possible as an effect of radiotherapy damage during prostate-cancer treatment

Keloid scarring and possible fatal urethral blockage in African and other black-skinned victims if penis is removed by surgery or trauma

Increased life expectancy - the one bonus, but a bad outcome for those suffering from mental weakness or osteoporosis

Therapy Options

Testosterone-Replacement Therapy, HRT for MEN, can take several forms. Originally it was likely to be slow-release injections but these inevitably led to discomforting peaks and troughs.

Daily capsules are easier to take but today gels are more used, either in single doses for application to the skin or from pump dispensers. To my knowledge, no therapy allows for doses calibrated to the exact need of a man and his symptoms.

Optimal Testosterone Levels

The correct testosterone level for a man is not easy to agree, for age and innate levels should all be considered. As patients now have more ready access to their medical records, it's suggested they look to see where they are on the testosterone tests for which they have asked and then discuss this further with their doctor.

Until ways are found to make minor adjustments to testosterone levels, this remains a contentious matter, largely because 55+ men might want to achieve an 'average' testosterone level, when all their life they have had something rather less.

Perhaps levels of testosterone should regularly be measured from about the time all men are 55, so that false playing fields are not pursued in later life?

Risks of Self Dosing

In many countries testosterone is available via the web for self-medication but unsupervised ingestion can be very dangerous. Side effects can include rampant acne, stroke or heart ailments and a degree of priapism, particularly when used in conjunction with corrective drugs for erectile dysfunction.

Universally these problems are caused by unsupervised overdosing or because patients have other compromised organ functions. Sometimes, the symptoms thought to be testosterone related are nothing of the kind and might be either neurotic or genuine mental issues.

Supervised, professional prescriptions would stop this, yet I have sympathy for many of those who self-medicate because their doctors will not. Few self-prescribers want to be super men, not even virile super men but hoped only to be returned to what they were, again to be dignified, capable, independent, and yes, sexual men.

PART FOUR

What Testosterone-Poverty Did To Me

A Future in Doubt

I was 58 when I was diagnosed with prostate cancer.

The discovery seemed an extraordinary blessing, because I had just returned to New Zealand after 30 years in the UK and four in Australia. A smart GP said 'I don't know who you are, so I am going to test for everything'.

Few GPs would have included the PSA test for prostate cancer for someone my age. The average age for diagnosis is between 65 and 69. If the doctor had not done the PSA blood test, it's very likely I'd be dead and unpleasantly so. That was the blessing. The discovery of cancer was equally a severe blow because I needed all my strength and wits to begin a new life, to start a new career.

Suddenly my future was in doubt, in every way.

Possibilities Destroyed

Few doctors seem to believe a man of 58 can have a malignant prostate tumour and so do not regularly prescribe the PSA test, thus many if not most tumours are simply not discovered until it is too late, which inevitably means the condition is fatal.

Compared to the tell-tale lumps that publish the presence of breast cancer, prostate tumours grow to a dangerous state without immediately identifiable symptoms. Urinary problems are easily ignored, perhaps accepted as part of growing old; bone pains too are dismissed but are a sign that tumours have spread beyond the prostate, making it very difficult to treat. One way or another it is common for prostate cancer to be discovered so late that it is untreatable. Death is the inevitable result.

This pitiless lack of warning symptoms is the major factor in more men dying of prostate cancer than women died of breast cancer in 2018 and is why organised regular PSA testing for prostate cancer should be as common as breast cancer tests are for women.

The jeopardy most commonly cited for younger men with a tumour is that comparatively higher testosterone levels will make his cancer grow faster. The less-known and less-acknowledged peril is that the higher a man's testosterone level the more extreme his reactions will be to the sudden chemical removal of the hormone as preparation for treatment, something confirmed publically in my case by a Daily Mail article quoted later in this section.

Once tests confirmed a fast-growing malignant prostate tumour I had to choose between treatment by radiotherapy or by radical surgery, which removes the prostate entirely but is likely to create impotency and I didn't want to give up penile pleasures if this could be avoided. Partial removal of the prostate might not have been any better because the pathways of the very fine nerves that control erections travel over the back of the prostate. It is immensely difficult to guarantee they will not be severed or damaged. The slightest damage affects erectile ability, and complete severance means a man can never have a natural erection again.

If you are a private (rich) patient, especially in the United States, there's a strong chance those nerves can be saved by a specialist surgeon and a man will then continue to have full erections, even if all his prostate is removed.

The burning effects of radiotherapy can also damage those erectile nerves, so unless a millionaire, all men diagnosed with prostate-cancer must face up to the possibility of permanently impeded or destroyed erectile possibilities.

Incontinence Fears

At the time, medics in NZ were not permitted to make treatment recommendations. To complicate the pressure of deciding what I wanted to do, I had the usual pathetic worries about DRE, the digital rectal examination necessary to examine the prostate, establishing if it is smooth, hard and healthy or if it is lumpy and cancerous or otherwise unwell.

Was I clean internally? What about stories that a finger touching your prostate can promote an erection? Is it true this is a way you can tell if a man is gay or not? Might I break wind at the wrong time and if so would a disgusting baked-bean pong still be hanging around?

These and other fears are what prevent millions of men having an examination that might save their lives. And these are the fears that women must tell a man to get over – to save his life.

A digital rectal examination takes seconds, so erections are unlikely and anyway the examiner is concentrating on your other side. Neither do you leave the surgery wearing a sign on your forehead that someone has just had a finger up your bum. What is true is that those few seconds of digital intrusion might well have helped saved you from a particularly painful and distressing death.

'I notice no-one ever thinks about the poor buggers who have to do it' I said to my GP as he was washing his hands.

'Don't worry about me,' he smirked, 'I get paid for it!'

Every type of radiotherapy for prostate-cancer treatment has nasty possible side effects, particularly of bladder or bowel incontinence and I particularly worried about the latter. If you ask, the chances of incontinence create much more anguish in prostate-cancer patients than possible loss of virility but this is rarely addressed, pre-treatment or after it. Bowel incontinence seems to be dismissed as a minor side-effect of radiotherapy and yet is one of the most enduring and life-changing.

Avoiding the Truth with a Grunt

Oncologist Dr Brown (not his real name) at Auckland City Hospital told me I did not qualify for the British Medical Research Council Trial he was leading. Yet on the second consultation, when I had to decide on my treatment, I was offered a place on the trial, and urged to accept, for reasons never explained.

My brother Bruce had accompanied me, knowing I was frightened by the cancer diagnosis and was thus likely to be confused or not remember or understand what was said to me. We heard about testosterone-suppression therapy for the first time, which I easily understood to mean a chemical castration. It was touted as necessary because it would stop prostate-tumour growth, which would make the plotting of treatment by radiotherapy more focussed and thus more assured, as indeed it was.

I was told to expect side-effects of hot flushes, lowered libido and reduced erectile ability from the hormone suppression. I then asked how long the effect of this chemical castration lasted, a question based on my knowledge of some possible effects of testosterone loss, learned through research for a proposed novel featuring history's eunuchs. My specific question was, 'Does it just switch back after the radiotherapy?'

Dr Brown answered with a grunt.

Not with a single word.

Just a grunt, with an upwards inflection.

My brother and I had no way of knowing this was not an assent but a prevarication with profound implications that would affect the rest of my life. In the careful wording of the later legal challenges I pursued, Dr Brown had not 'properly warned' me of the possible effects of testosterone suppression.

He didn't explain that the testosterone suppression might take two years to reverse naturally. He definitely did not tell us that sometimes the body's testosterone-making function never recovers. He certainly did not mention a single one of the many other possible side-effects, including those of the radiotherapy.

My brother made a sworn statement that I was thus not 'properly warned'. This, together with my submissions, was utterly dismissed when I pursued my case for Medical Misadventure in a New Zealand system famously weighted against complainants.

If I had known the truth I could have refused hormone treatment and chosen radiotherapy without it, or discussed that option anyway. My life would have been greatly different and I still wonder if the doctor was suddenly desperate for a final patient on the BMRC trial.

Effects Before Radiotherapy Began

At the time, I was elated. Although growing quite fast, the cancer was early and small and I was being treated at what many told me is one of the best Oncology clinics in the world, certainly in the Southern hemisphere, and I was taking part in a trial prepared by Britain's august Medical Research Council; it seemed to be the Rolls-Royce of care and certainty.

Treatment of my tumour began late in August with a first painful, abdominal implant of Zoladex (goserelin), the drug chosen to suppress my testosterone. In less than a week hot flushes came without warning and stayed without compassion, sometimes for three or four hours at a time. Mercifully they were rarely at night. Erections ceased and I empathised with the wistful looks of those much older men who sat on benches and watched the potent pass by. Three months later, I had the second implant, just before radiotherapy began. This time it didn't hurt as much, but the next day I was depressed.

Twice during the three previous years a black dog of depression, as Churchill called it, had firmly attached itself to me. Both times I had recognised the problem and both times drug treatment and counselling had worked quickly. I thought it a blessing that I was stable at the time of my diagnosis and that coping with cancer hadn't caused a relapse into depression.

The bout of depression after the second implant wasn't extreme, only lasted a few days and seemed clearly associated with that, perhaps a reaction to the extreme pain of the procedure. The effect shouldn't have been the sudden rush of suppressive drug, because it was a slow-release system. I forgot about it and radiotherapy began five days a week in the first days of December.

No Response, No Touchy-Feely

At the end of December, just after Christmas, I had a third Zoladex implant. This time the pain and my reaction was so severe it took an hour for me to recover. A few days later I woke in a state of such extreme depression it was like living in a bowl of wet cement, with every move and thought slowed, inhibited and weighted down. I was frightened by the severity and depth of my mental state and so, unusually for me, I recognised that I needed to ask for help.

It was a Friday afternoon. A sympathetic hospital-staff psychiatrist agreed I was severely depressed and said he would contact the Taylor Centre, a Government-funded centre for mental health, and that they would be in touch over the weekend. But they weren't. Now doubly incontinent and sleeping badly, both predicated reactions to the radiotherapy, I was so incapable of normal life that for those days I ate only what a finger and thumb pulled off a loaf of bread.

I didn't hear from the Taylor Centre, yet I dared not call them in case this confirmed my twisted, depressed thinking that I wasn't worth their interest. Subsequently, the New Year, and my New Year's Day birthday passed in a frightened, sad, hungry torpor, racked by hot flushes and often painful twin incontinences. I heard myself thinking that I'd rather be dying of the cancer, for at least there would be an end to the horrors. Suicide was seen as a close and welcome relief.

When radiotherapy treatment began again on Monday, there was still no follow up by the Oncology department's psychiatrist, no mention by anyone of my asking for help and still nothing from the Taylor Centre. I was confirmed in my view I wasn't sick enough to be bothered with. When I looked around the hospital corridors this was easy to understand. Boys and girls, hairless and colourless, were always somewhere seen, silently wheeled by on trolleys. Grey mothers with frightened children were, too, or fathers who had never before been sick, hating to need help from children with whom they had never had a proper conversation.

All these seemed to deserve attention more than me.

I've been very independent all my life and I reluctantly accepted that once more I would have to, well, just get on with it. Yet, in the touchy-feely world of modern medicine there were brochures and posters everywhere telling me what I knew viscerally, that the quality of my care should have been better.

It's What You Remember That Counts

By Wednesday the depression lifted. I put the episode to one side. In a few weeks I would be finished with the radiotherapy.

Eventually, I mentioned the lack of Taylor Centre follow-up during a routine weekly session with a hospital doctor. Even today her answer floors me.

Rather than promising to check what had happened, she said

I should write to the Taylor Centre. Write to them! This to a cancer patient towards the end of physically disruptive radiotherapy and who's just complained of severe depression, of feeling suicidal and of a request for help not being followed up, of being isolated over a full weekend? I didn't have the strength to protest, but it confirmed my warped view I was just a time waster in the hospital's opinion. It didn't seem possible this was modern hospital practice, that she was properly doing her job with proper care and compassion, so I judged that somehow the fault must only have been mine.

When radiotherapy finished in mid-January I remember walking out with a huge smile on my face. It was a glorious midsummer day, and the balmy shadows of the trees encouragingly soothed my hot flushes. I didn't have a hair of the dog of depression, and the cancer was almost certainly zapped.

Life Could Only Get Better

Of course it was going to seem worse for a while, as reaction to radiotherapy began to dig in. There was a peculiar type of tiredness that made the body leaden. Bladder and bowel incontinence caused by internal burning by radiotherapy continued to mean double leakage and control issues; I had been given no advice about or supplies of absorbent pads. Leaving the house to shop for food and staples was a nightmare of clenched muscles and, sometimes, shame.

With minimised embarrassment and maximum solitariness I managed, believing the more I lived something like a normal life, the faster normality would return. And hadn't Dr Brown said the effects of the testosterone suppression would revert once radiotherapy was over? That would make it easier to cope with the radiotherapy side effects, wouldn't it? Well, he had grunted, rather than said this but that belief was the only beacon I had and my gaze was fixed on this single beam of hope and recovery.

I had not kept notes day-to-day after diagnosis, as I had been urged, because my travel and food-writing careers in London had been based on an opposite path. When Prudence Glynn relinquished her heady post as Fashion Editor of The Times, she was to be succeeded by Suzy Menkes. They went together to the Haute Couture Collections in Paris and as the first show began Suzy Menkes took out a pad and pen, only to have them taken away.

'It's what you remember that counts,' Prudence Glynn said.

Thus, I took no contemporary notes but soon after wrote summaries of what happened to support my appeals for financial compensation – as the brochures said I should; those summaries are the basis of what you now read.

A Lurch into Feminising

By mid-February I was suffering badly from sleep deprivation and incontinence that was sometimes cramping and sore but when the Oncology nurse rang each week I said I was doing ok. I expected and asked for nothing, to protect myself from further disappointment.

Then something frightening happened. When towelling myself dry after a shower I noticed leg hair coming off. I rubbed at my chest, and then my arms.

That hair came off too. When I went to shave I realised my beard had softened.

Body-hair loss wasn't a symptom I had been told to expect. I wasn't on chemotherapy, so it couldn't be side-effects of that and anyway my head hair was intact. With a nauseated lurch I understood that, rather than lifting, the hormone suppression was consolidating. I was not getting better but worse. The hormone therapy wasn't reverting as Dr Brown has grunted it would.

A bubble of self-deceit then burst. I had been ignoring other disturbing physical and mental changes. I had accommodated or ignored them because I believed, needed to believe, I was getting over the testosterone suppression and would soon be over the radiotherapy.

My symptoms told me I was a testosterone-free eunuch, a Testosterone-Pauper, when I should have been on my way to being a whole man again. When I should have been masculinising again, I was feminising.

Abandoned

Patients have a charter in New Zealand from both the Health and Disability Commissioner, whose job is to apportion blame where there is a breakdown of procedure, and from the Accident Compensation Corporation, who agree compensation. These charters seek to guarantee patients are treated with dignity, that they know the name of the people who are dealing with their case, and that they are involved in all discussions of diagnosis and of suggested treatment; there is a distinct requirement that not only should patients be involved, but should be seen to understand and to agree with what is suggested.

I finished my radiotherapy at Auckland City Hospital with no care plan and with no explanation of what to expect or not to expect. In retrospect, I believe the oncology staff were more experienced at dealing with older patients, whose testosterone levels before suppression were much lower than mine had been. Those older patients generally have fewer side effects of testosterone suppression and so perhaps severe reactions like mine were simply beyond the experience, the care-skills or knowledge-pool of the department.

Maps to Nowhere

The symptoms I had ignored but then acknowledged make chilling reading, yet they will be no surprise to many other prostate-cancer patients who have been on hormone-suppression therapy, particularly those who are relatively younger.

The side-effects of testosterone suppression and their range and depth are impossible to predict; there is no pattern of symptoms and nothing to help know that if you suffer one you will suffer another. There are no rules

Just as some women sail through menopause, some men will notice little difference to daily life if their testosterone is removed. Once I had full cognition of what was happening to me I still struggled to believe it, thinking of those stock-character women in TV comedies who so readily tell you, 'the doctor said he'd never seen anything like it – biggest he'd ever seen etc etc'. Later I found my symptoms were indeed unusually profound and wide-ranging. Thus, I was right to feel I should have had more care.

No Salvation

I would never have agreed to the testosterone suppression by Zoladex if I had been told of the full possibility of side effects from testosterone suppression, and that it could take two years to revert, if it reverted at all.

In those days oncologists believed what the drug manufacturers told them (Astra Zeneca in this case), who were adamant that drugs such as Zoladex had no effect on mood and depression. Even today the admitting of this is minimal on packaging and in advice to prospective radiotherapy patients.

Now I know why old men, who have lost testosterone by natural depletion, can be so confused and helpless. Yet, they have had time to adjust as normal life slowly ebbed away. Testosterone-suppression victims have it ripped from them.

Did I have friends and family? Well, yes, but I couldn't tell them everything, and those I did tell didn't understand everything. How could they? Anyway, they had their lives to live and, as I had once done, all of them universally believed that I would be well looked after by the hospital and by the specialist teams there.

Yes, I often wanted to kill myself. All that stopped me was the unshakeable knowledge that what was happening was not normal. I wasn't going to be a victim of other people's disinterest.

I arranged an emergency consultation with Dr Brown.

Gross Humiliation

The meeting was on March 7th, 2001. By now I was in the deepest phase of the debilitating reaction to radiotherapy, exceptionally sleep deprived, and overwhelmed by the conscious realisation of my physical and mental disabilities, about none of which I had been warned. I was fragile, utterly exhausted and, most of all, because I was finally admitting something was seriously wrong, I was emotionally naked. The possibility of subterfuge was over. Stupidly, I did not arrange someone independent to come with me, thinking that my need for help would be plain and acknowledged.

When I went into the consulting room accompanied by the sympathetic Trials Co-ordinator, a plump woman without any sort of uniform was already seated with folded arms by the curtained examination area. I was never introduced to her, a direct contravention of what is supposed to happen. As he sat down opposite me, Dr Brown first mumbled 'It's never happened before, never happened before'.

I took this as a good thing, believing that when a doctor recognises a problem is new or serious he or she will feel validated by the challenge, that this is what their expertise is most properly aimed at resolving.

After a brief chat Dr Brown said he would examine me and soon I was on a table, with underpants down for a DRE. I didn't really understand the need for this and also sensed Dr Brown was curiously anxious and dithery. I took the opportunity to point out I had fat around my hips, something that had never happened to me before. I still believe that as he first probed me and then prodded my hips Dr Brown was mumbling: menopause, menopause.

I couldn't ask Dr Brown what he meant. In my state of self-doubt I simply accepted that he didn't feel it worthwhile communicating with me. However, I am perfectly happy to discount what I believe Dr Brown said, because it is what he next did that matters rather more, that injured me more profoundly.

Dr Brown left the examination cubicle without a word and then began a low conversation with the Trials Co-ordinator and, I think, another woman who had come into the consulting room. I lay there abandoned on an examination table, like a dirty cup on a sink bench. It was grossly humiliating. I was fragile, lying with my pants down, in a cubicle with the curtain that had been left half open. I had a slimy arse after being digitally penetrated, was still tormented by hideous hot flushes, still didn't know for sure what might be wrong with me or what might be done about it.

I had to shout, to ask if it was all right for me to get dressed and to come out, like a child begging for an end to a punishment but much more shaming.

Worse was to come.

Three Months?

After prescribing something to settle the burning pain of urination, which would also reduce the frequency, Dr Brown quickly dismissed my question about testosterone replacement by saying this was impossible because it might regenerate the prostate cancer. That was it. There was no acknowledgement of a connection between my fallen mood, no interest in any of my other symptoms, and once again no honest, helpful prognosis of how long these might continue. There was nothing that could be done, and that was that. Brown, as a radiology oncologist, clearly felt that his job was completed. I was too overwhelmed to argue my case further. I was struggling to dam tears I knew would never stop.

Anxious for something concrete out of the meeting I then had to ask three times to get a form for a blood test, just to confirm where my testosterone level might be, because if it were rising that would be encouraging. Once the blood-test request was reluctantly signed I had to force an answer about who would tell me the results.

Then Dr Brown delivered his final wound. He murmured that he would see me in three months. He was abandoning me a second time, this time without a single straw of hope, comfort or sympathy and for three months. Dr Brown clearly thought that whatever was wrong with me was so minor, so unimportant – perhaps even deserved - that I should stop complaining and simply disappear for three months. It seemed like contempt from the one person whom I expected to give me more care, not less.

Perhaps Dr Brown felt that having cured the tumour he had no other responsibility to me? That wasn't the quality of care I saw promised on every wall of the hospital.

Emergency Tears

Next morning I had a call from the Taylor Centre, apologising for not responding to the earlier request for help and leaving me a contact number because I had been referred to them for further support. The Taylor Centre treats sick minds, so it appeared I was thought of only as mentally deficient in some way, that I had a mental problem un-associated with testosterone suppression. Today, this seems to have been a neat but nasty way of deflecting attention and responsibility. If a surgeon finds something unexpected during an operation, he must identify and solve that and I still believe that is what an oncologist should do, too.

After this meeting I could do little at home but stand or sit in clotted silence, buried alive in hopeless incomprehension of what the next months might hold with no offer of support or care other than referral to a mental facility.

That night, as I was telling the story to a visitor the tears finally began. I knew they wouldn't stop, and I used the emergency number left by the Taylor Centre.

A Cannonball Broadside

This time, someone was there in an hour and I sobbed my story, of just wanting help, wanting to talk about getting some of my testosterone back, regardless of any cancerous risk. I cared little for danger to my body; it was the injuries to my mind that I wanted fixed. I needed to be able to earn a living, to be independent again.

I was put to bed with heavy sleeping tablets and the next day all sorts of welcome support appeared: a continence nurse, social worker and more, but I had no idea if they were there because of Dr Brown or of the Taylor Centre. The social worker had worked with Dr Brown and sympathised fully. She said: 'He's just not treating the whole patient'. She tried to speak to Dr Brown on my behalf but never once got through to him. Her wisdom was greatly needed but never recognised.

The support was not on-going and I now wonder why some sort of regular visit or a degree of home help was never offered; it was certainly needed. The radiotherapy-related symptoms began to ease, but the testosterone-suppression symptoms got worse. Or perhaps I now had a clearer window through which to see them?

Some days later the Trials Co-ordinator telephoned to say my testosterone count was castrate level, barely able to be measured. Absorbing this as proof of my plight I asked if there shouldn't be some sort of treatment plan, some goal to be working towards to give me that 'best possible Quality of Life' I was promised so fulsomely in the brochures and posters.

She offered the chance to speak to Dr Brown. When I had done this once before, I found his foreign accent difficult to understand on the telephone, something I expected was as embarrassing to him as to me. I needed clarity but I didn't want to fight for it, or get it wrong, or unintentionally upset the doctor. Yet, when I explained why I'd rather not speak to Dr Brown, thinking this was respectful, it was interpreted by him as a refusal to speak to him, a personal insult when it was quite the reverse.

The Trials Co-ordinator was completely sympathetic to the problem, saying she understood this situation from past experience, and as an alternative put me in touch with another specialist, whom I will call Dr White. He was the first to tell me that testosterone suppression doesn't just flick back after radiotherapy as it had been grunted it might. It could take as much as two years. He added that sometimes testosterone doesn't come back at all.

It was like being broadsided by cannonballs.

The Last Flickers Extinguished

My greatest thought was wonderment that Dr Brown had withheld the truth. Perhaps he knew everything about radiotherapy but didn't know enough about testosterone suppression? Whatever the truth, I had been sentenced not to know if or when I would ever be back to normal again, whether or not I would ever be able to count or drive, park, find my way, ever be able to work and earn again . . . Rather than the best possible Quality of Life, it seemed I was to have none.

In Dr White's follow-up letter to Dr Brown he indicated a slightly lesser time span but two years is what he said to me: perhaps he included prep and radiotherapy time. He gave a number of possible reasons for my symptoms, but put hormone suppression at the end, as the least likely. Depression, he said was one likely cause of my symptoms but he did not connect this to the hormone-suppression treatment.

Subsequently Dr White had the unfounded audacity to suggest I wanted my testosterone back for the sake of sexual life. I knew I had never once mentioned this. It was deeply insulting, a snide diminishment of me as an individual and a dismissal of what I was suffering. What does it say about him?

I felt a double betrayal of not being properly warned about a possible two-year or longer wait for the return of my testosterone and then of no proper intermediate care and support for my very apparent side-effect symptoms. The last flickers of strength and self-regard I harboured were extinguished. It's still impossible to find the words that would accurately describe the sense of isolation and of being treated at every turn as someone utterly without value or individuality.

This time, true clinical depression added its black weight and fiercely shackled me in terrible bondage. And I was still without testosterone.

Marooned

Spatial ability is about the judging of distance, the abstract understanding of volume, the instinctive calculation of speed, the ability to convert maps into reality and to get where you want. My spatial senses disappeared almost totally.

I found it increasingly hard to drive safely, and began to drive only by day and only when there was a desperate need. All my life I had done the map reading when routes had to be planned or would often accurately find my way by instinct. Whether in cities or the bush, getting lost simply wasn't an option.

Now I spent hours, with a map in my hand, looking fruitlessly for places I had been to before. It did little for self-esteem to telephone baffled hosts saying I couldn't find my way to them. I never admitted to anyone that I was not certain I would be able to get myself home.

Three times I escaped a serious car accident by centimetres because I was not able accurately to assess distances or speeds. Parking, a skill about which I had justifiably boasted, became impossible. My car was increasingly battered and scratched and in supermarket car parks I would find myself walking past my awkwardly or dangerously parked car again and again, until I felt no one would see me getting back in to it. When I got home, parking close to the kerb was simply beyond me, time after time.

I was finding going up and down stairs a dangerous challenge, for without a sense of space it is easy to misjudge steps and then to stumble, up or down. Getting on to an escalator became as challenging as doing a Times crossword without a pen. Sometimes I was marooned for ages, not trusting myself to stairs or escalator until some survivalist dignity could be accessed. All the while hoping the bladder and the bowels would hold.

Everything to do with counting or mental calculation ground to a halt. I became utterly confused by anything mathematical and could no longer understand money or mathematics or calculate in my head, when once what used to be called Mental Arithmetic had been a special skill.

Like Blanche Dubois in A Streetcar Named Desire, I was commonly grateful for the kindness of strangers, reduced to offering money in an extended palm and hoping the shop assistant was honest. I couldn't count out cash or coins because the figures tumbled from my head and could not be retrieved. When a pharmacist asked me how many of a drug I still had at home, my mind refused to work. I flushed with heat and then, frustrated, ashamed, defeated, I burst into tears. I bless him for whisking me out into the back of his shop, away from gaping customers, and for never mentioning it again.

The worst of this inability to calculate mentally meant I could no longer create recipes, the basis of my career since 1974, when I co-partnered the opening of Mr Christian's, a delicatessen just off London's famous Portobello Road. This meant the catastrophic loss of a major book commission, a book based on sensible eating to help prevent cancer and based on impeccable international research from the United States, a project that might have given me a firmer financial platform for later life.

The very basis of my UK career on television, radio and in publishing had disappeared. The most obvious way I could have regained financial stability and self-esteem in New Zealand was denied.

Too Close to Madness

As things worsened, I suffered grossly from word loss in speech. I would simply hit barriers and no word would come, not even alternatives. It is a horrible feeling, like being only half alive.

On the morning my publisher came finally to discuss what would happen about the book I could no longer write, I burst into tears because like an untongued infant I could not remember or say the word 'sink' even though I was looking at it and pointing at it. Infants have my sympathy for their rages when no one understands what they want.

At worst I forgot my name, and thus how to write my signature when signing a cheque or for goods bought on credit. Imagine standing in a queue with only half a signature done - and not knowing what comes next. And then going into a major hot flush before it finally came, if it came at all. More than once the loss was so profound I could not retrieve my signature and so had to switch to an EFTPOS direct debit card, for I had my code written inside my wallet. No touchless cards to help the afflicted then.

Of course, if this were to be a day when I had not taken care of my clothes and hadn't shaved for a few days, few of the looks I got were sympathetic. Until I saw fear, disgust and disdain in the eyes of other people I had no sense of what I looked like. I wouldn't see I hadn't shaved for days or recognise I was wearing clothes I had slept in more than once. When almost everything that marks out your identity has been taken from you, clothes and appearance make no sense.

It is common to put something into the microwave when you mean to put it into the refrigerator. But I would do it four times in a row and then, not being able to remember or know what I wanted to do, burst into awful childlike tears of incomprehension. Then I'd do it wrong again. It was too close to madness, and a hastened death seemed the only way out.

It is chilling to think most of this was avoidable.

Taking Them On

There was grateful confirmation from within the family that my symptoms were indeed related to testosterone loss.

Not long before, my brother Bruce had realised his memory was failing him badly. Facts, telephone numbers, dates and appointments he once remembered with great facility were lost to him and he was also depressed. It took a long time to discover the cause was Testosterone-Poverty and how this had happened.

Bruce had had a tumour on his pituitary gland. In a curious stroke that might be called lucky, the tumour had twisted and choked itself to death, but not before destroying the part of the pituitary gland that controls the manufacture of testosterone. Testosterone-Replacement Therapy had then helped him regain his memory and his ability to work and to earn and still does.

I realised then that those who had chemically castrated me in New Zealand did not know that the effects of low-testosterone levels and of testosterone suppression were being looked at more carefully in other parts of the world. I felt I had to challenge this dearth and it didn't frighten me to do this. Fear is one of man's greatest stimulants and I was profoundly afraid of a frail and pointless future, a sentence to be on the outskirts of life forever more. Anyway, I had taken on received opinion before.

Roads Less-Well Travelled

The third book I wrote was BREAD and YEAST-COOKERY (Macdonald Educational 1978), and the very superior consultant to whom it was given was rather sniffy and wanted changes I knew were wrong. I prevailed; she apologised and said she had learned a lot. Later Elizabeth David wrote it was one of the few books on the subject that was accurate and worth owning.

In 1980 I'd led an expedition to Pitcairn Island and then written FRAGILE PARADISE, still the only biography of Fletcher Christian, my great-great-great-great grandfather. Because the mutiny on BOUNTY was not that of a ship but of one man against another it was the first time it was possible to pit Christian and Bligh against one another as rounded characters rather than as figments.

I discovered a huge amount of original material, yet when my project was first mooted I was told that if there were no Fletcher Christian biography it was because there was no evidence on which to base one. A rather famed London agent thought no-one would be interested in 'the fate of some 18th-century sailor'.

I'd stuck to many solitary guns in my television and writing career, too. Professional chefs mocked when I first demonstrated non-stick pans on BBC-TV's Breakfast Time, but now only chippies cook without them. I raged against the hydrogenated oils of 'spreads', recommending pure, better-tasting butter, and now their trans-fatty acids are proven to be more dangerous. I've campaigned about the inclusion of acidic, under-cooked onion in anything, mocked the self-assessed and often unproven righteousness of organics, refused to join the tasteless battalions of quick-fix writers, who once put cheese onto every dish and 'popped it under the grill until bubbling and golden brown' and who now put chilli into everything.

That's still my favourite hobby horse, the misuse of chilli. Chilli is not a flavouring but mouth trauma, a sensation that negates everything wondrous about eating unless you are very poor. The heat of chillies was once the refuge of the most underprivileged, used most prolifically where Earth's bounty is least. The pain of the burned tongue creates feel-good endorphins, so even when eating rice with a few other scraps something seems to happen in the mouth and a good-feeling is engendered. Endorphin highs rather than good taste are what chillies give, and create genuine addiction, so that more and more are needed to feed that as well as to penetrate the burn-scarred taste buds.

I was used to being on roads less travelled. I determined to open 21st century eyes to the effects of Testosterone-Poverty on today's 55+ men's health.

Changes Made by Testosterone-Replacement

Telling my testosterone stories became the whisper-thin lifeline I threw myself, not for revenge or to be vindictive but to air the truth that the medical profession seems largely to know all about women's hormones but little about men's. Accepting I was getting no therapeutic care directly from the BRMC Trial and the Auckland City Hospital, I withdrew from both. The psychological help offered by regular visits to the Taylor Centre changed nothing because they were treating the wrong condition. The drugs made life more difficult than ever, including objects morphing into threatening ghouls, even when I was driving.

Yet even through the mental mist I knew that testosterone replacement would make a difference and months later I successfully fought for and won a referral to the same endocrinology practice that had helped my brother. The endocrinologist had no truck with the idea that Testosterone-Replacement Therapy might stimulate new cancer growth, agreeing that the right to a decent Quality of Life overrode this minor and unproven risk. He prescribed Testosterone-Replacement at once, with weekly blood tests to check both my testosterone and PSA levels. My PSA never rose and the cancer has not returned.

It took two weeks for the first sign that testosterone replacement was working. The erectile nerves had been permanently damaged but something close to normal function was slowly restored; it could have been very much worse.

It took years to get the mental effects of the suppression under control. First, I had to get rid of the clinical depression. Only after being referred to a psychiatric service where the practitioner interrupted, questioned and gave advice rather than sitting pompous and silent, as others had done, did I feel the black dog might stir itself and leave me. One day there was a click behind my right ear – it had gone. As my facilities came back, I discovered I could write again, as long as there were no recipes involved, but I was still anchored to my house because of the double incontinence about which very little had been done.

Justification Published

A difficult research trip back to London included enquiries direct to the Medical Research Council and others, who all agreed with my assessment of what had happened to me and to the lack of proper care.

It wasn't until years later that there was very public justification for what I believed had been a complete misunderstanding of testosterone suppression. In February 2009, The Daily Mail published a major article about my case.

Dr Harry Naerger, a consultant urologist at Frimley Park Hospital in Surrey is quoted as saying he was 'not surprised to hear that Glynn's life was so affected . . . if a man has a relatively high level of testosterone to begin with, then rapidly reducing it down to zero is far more likely to cause the side effects Glynn experienced'. Of all his patients reporting physical effects, around 5 per cent reported mood swings, irritableness and depression to varying degrees.

He added, 'There is also a groundswell of opinion that testosterone and brain function are closely linked,' he said. 'Not all the effects of reducing testosterone are apparent straight away, which can explain why Glynn's symptoms took months to develop and a long time to repair.'

For the full article, see: http://www.dailymail.co.uk/health/article-1153602/Hormone-jabs-saved-life-ruined-reveals-TV-chef-cancer victim.html#ixzz2cltFcuaa

But this was in the future and in another country.

Back in New Zealand I sued for Medical Misadventure but the system was unbalanced. Neither Dr Brown nor a responsible representative was ever present at a hearing and the authorities repeated ad nauseam, and without supporting evidence, that I had been 'properly warned'.

Eventually, I understood I had neither the money nor the will to keep fighting. How could I, when the authorities supposedly representing patients seemed so clearly biased in favour of the medical profession rather than in the pursuit of truth?

The only way I could protect what sanity I had regained, the only way I could profit from what skills were returning, was to sell up and return to London

The Price of Conviction

Socially, life was still difficult. I knew my mind wasn't yet totally secure but could be unfocussed or wander off target. Even so, I returned to work on QVC television and wrote HOW TO COOK WITHOUT RECIPES, both successfully. And then another disaster struck.

A relatively unknown side-effect of radiotherapy is that a sudden eruption of internal burn side-effects can flare up after a long period of relative calm. The time period is usually anything around ten years or 25 years. For me it was less than ten years. Double incontinence again struck with such vicious intent I was once more marooned. Eating became difficult and that made my general health suffer again, to say nothing of the daily mental anguish.

I was in a worse physical state than ever and soon had to withdraw from the food world, particularly from judging at the Great Taste Awards, which I had named. It was bad enough having to be there padded up back and front, which seemed wrong in the presence of food. The result of tasting so many foods in a day would also put me into bed for days. It was better to withdraw, and so yet another part of my identity was torn from me.

While more treatments for the new collapses of my bladder and bowels were tried and failed (don't say yes to botoxing your bladder!) the Testosterone- Replacement Therapy was at least working. Eventually a drug called *fesoterodine fumarate* gave me bladder control within 24 hours, begging the question why it had not been prescribed before.

I was capable of writing although I was aware that other times my mind was still far from normal in thinking. To cope with those other discomforts and the fears of unpredictable self-shaming, I pretty much stayed home alone for three years and wrote MRS CHRISTIAN - BOUNTY MUTINEER, telling the unknown story of my Tahitian great-great-great-great grandmother, Mauatua, a founding foremother of Pitcairn Island, which was first in the world to give women the vote and to make education compulsory for girls. I'm very proud to carry Mauatua's fighting blood and to have inherited Fletcher's demonstrated belief that social convictions might demand a high personal price.

Me – Not Them

My natural testosterone never returned, so for almost 20 years I have suffered Primary Hypo-gonadism. I would not be alive to write this book without daily Testosterone-Replacement Therapy and don't dare think what life would have been without this. I can't help wonder at the pain of those who had none.

Of course, I am grateful that I am alive because the prostate tumour was so successfully vanquished and of course I understand that the internal burning which still causes a great deal of discomfort and distress is integral to my survival.

Yet I can't forget that I had no help or encouragement to find what really made life possible for me again, that identity-saving Testosterone-Replacement Therapy. It was my efforts and insistence, my native-born grit and determination not to be the victim of neglect that saved me.

It was me who rescued my mind, my identity and my future, not any care and compassion from those who suppressed my testosterone and who then dismissed themselves from any responsibility for the awful and many side-effects. I had slowly hauled myself up to claim my right to a decent Quality of Life again, wanting victory rather than to succumb to victimhood.

Writing helped but it became apparent that I needed to do more than that to be Glynn Christian again. I created and taught a semester about taste and flavour for Drexel University of Philadelphia, Pa, at their London campus. I also became a guide at the Victoria and Albert Museum. The slowly restored abilities resulting from Testosterone-Replacement Therapy are what made these possible, but the ill-health and anguish caused by the incontinences meant I had to give up both.

The last of my skills that returned after many years' absence was being a creative cook and that was the one that most helped me feel I was me again, yet I know I still make dreadful mistakes.

Even so, the dietary inhibitions that hoped to help with the digestive complications caused by constant bowel problems made entertaining and being entertained increasingly challenging. Both almost ceased, isolating me further.

Shouting for a Better World

In an honest and fair world I should have been able successfully to sue in New Zealand for Medical Misadventure and they authorities might have learned something. This was prevented by what seemed to be a misunderstanding of the possible effects of testosterone-suppression in both Auckland City Hospital and the Health and Disability Commissioner's office and what appeared to me to be an unwillingness to engage in discussion or further education.

Now, the many years of misery and hardship mean that, rather than the comfortable and financially self-sufficient old-age I had worked for, I am a State Pensioner who needs Housing Benefit. I couldn't be more grateful to Wandsworth Council and HM Government for helping keep me safe, secure and warm. More important are my few loyal and supportive friends, who until now will have known little.

Whenever I feel blue or disenchanted with my life I only have to look about to see how many are much worse off than me, physically and mentally, yet can't help thinking of how things might have been, what I might have been able to do if testosterone loss had not been permitted to take such a hold on me but had been replaced soon after the radiotherapy treatment ended.

Recently, a colo-rectal specialist in London told me that he was 'painfully aware' that too many treatments are given without real thought for their side effects by those who prescribed them. It was an effect, he thought, caused by such huge caseloads that patients become mere numbers and exercises rather than people, no longer valued as individuals whose life and Quality of Life are held in doctors' and specialists' hands.

That's even more reason for women and men to shout about Testosterone-Replacement Therapy and to be certain they are heard above the crowds, to make both ordinary people and the medical profession understand and implement The HRT for MEN Imperatives.

Most men and women do not know Testosterone-Replacement Therapy is possible, is 'a thing', and many of those men would not seek it, simply because they are men and thus likely to be reticent, embarrassed or just plain stubborn.

Please be certain that no man has to be special to suffer the effects of Testosterone-Poverty. They can be shopkeepers or peers, taxi drivers or truck fleet owners, train guards or street cleaners, clerks, managers, MDs, MPs, COEs, chefs, waiters or security guards, writers, presenters, artists, rappers or jockeys. Or me. Or you.

Heightened awareness will encourage and inform others, both inside and outside the medical profession, and then help make HRT as common for men as it is for women. Testosterone-Replacement Therapy internationally could annually help improve the lives of hundreds of thousands of living men and of their families, friends and colleagues.

What a better world that would be.

In the meantime . . .

PART FIVE

The Six Types of Testosterone-Pauper

I: Age-related
II: Prostate Cancer
III: Chemical
IV: Trauma
V: Hero
VI: Disease or Disorder-related

I: Age-Related Testosterone-Paupers

Age-related Testosterone-Paupers are the most common sufferers of Testosterone-Poverty and each is an unwitting victim.

Insufferably, sneaky Nature relentlessly decreases a man's testosterone levels as he ages, wherever he lives in the world. By 60 he might have only 50% of his younger levels, whatever they were, high or low.

Then it continues to lessen.

If recognised, the condition is known medically as androgen-deficiency because it is not always full Hypo-gonadism. If the symptoms are specially severe it might these days be called the Male Andropause but it is nothing like a pause. Specialists in the condition are rare and are called andrologists. Men who have successfully sought help are more usually treated by endocrinologists, general specialists in hormones. Testosterone should be one of these hormones but in my experience endocrinologists can know and care much more about women's hormones than those of themselves and of other men.

Lowered interest in sex is an obvious and commonly accepted symptom. The many other effects (See: A Catechism of Testosterone Poverty) might not occur at all in some men or reduce so slowly that a man will adjust to them unthinkingly, accepting the diminishments as an inescapable part of growing old and not feeling his style or Quality of Life is affected.

Those are the lucky ones. They are doubly lucky in a curious way if diagnosed with prostate cancer, because it seems that the lower your testosterone level at the time, the fewer side-effects you might suffer when the testosterone is removed.

Testosterone-Poverty is an increasingly accepted reason why a once happy and capable man is depressed and bad tempered, a state complicated by the sex he no longer wants and can no longer do. The connection between low testosterone and altered mood or depression in 55+ men is more and more discussed, including in such as the august Journal of the British Medical Association (BMA), yet nothing seems to be done to make Testosterone-Replacement Therapy part of basic medical training and practice

Most men die with one or more of the several types of prostate-cancer that do not threaten their life. Those that die of prostate cancer and complications inevitably do so because the disease has no symptoms until it is too late to treat; thus the importance of regular PSA tests for every man 55+.

Punished Just for Growing Old

The effects of the slow, natural fade of testosterone levels can be ignored for only so long as a man ages. Then comes the dread day of an avoidable car accident, unnecessary upset by minor occurrences, increased rage at reduced numerate or spatial abilities, an inability to judge golf shots, or a breakdown of professional abilities, or the onset of osteoporosis and the inevitable curtailment of life that follows any of these.

Or a descent into wretchedness, tearfulness even.

Few GPs suspect lowered testosterone as a possible cause, generally diagnosing as depression, but testosterone levels are checked with a routine blood test that spots a weakness at once. This medical shortcoming is what destroys the life and loves of so many 55+ men in every country of the world. And that's largely because the phenomenon of a wide spectrum of men who live more than 60 years is quite new.

In 1891 the average life expectancy for men in the UK was just over 44 years. Upper-class men had the best health and would generally live rather longer but there were too few of them markedly to skew the statistics. Anecdotally there have also been fewer, less-privileged, rural men who triumphed and reached three-score-and-ten years or many more.

During the 1900s, longer life for the average UK man eventually worked its way down the population thanks to improved diet and working conditions and better treatment for everything from 'blood-poisoning' to cancer and heart conditions.

Domestic refrigeration is also credited with a major contribution, as this reduced the amount of mouldy food eaten.

The United Kingdom's Office for National Statistics says that in 1950 the average age at which men died had increased by over 20 years to about 66; 50 years later at the start of the new millennium it was 76 and it is increasing.

Physicians and endocrinologists must make a determined effort to recognise the link between these new levels of increased age and the effects of testosterone decline. In most men the effects are likely first to be noticeable once a man is approaching 60. It's obvious they will become even more pronounced the longer a man lives; modern medicines he is taking, malnutrition and high alcohol intake can also contribute to his descent into Testosterone-Poverty.

No Case Studies

For millennia much could have been learned about the effects of Testosterone-Poverty by simple observation of both pre-pubertal and adult-made eunuchs, but the abundant source of case studies for long-term complete Testosterone-Poverty was lost to us because no-one understood the specific role played by testosterone.

Testosterone was first isolated only in 1935, when there were few adult-made eunuchs alive. Photographs of some of the last eunuchs employed in The Forbidden City showed many had grown bosoms and records show they usually lived longer than whole men but the pathology that created these ex-men was quite unknown.

Modern men are being punished just because they have grown old and because modern medicine has not kept up to date with what this super-aging means to the male mind and body. This is why there is not a deep catalogue for the medical profession's reference or education.

Without centuries of case studies on file, as there are for women's hormones and menopause, general practitioners can't recognise testosterone-loss as the likely cause of mind and body symptoms of ageing men and thus can't or won't treat them with Testosterone-Replacement Therapy that would greatly improve victims' Quality of Life, as well as that of those around them.

Public 'Men' Things

A common, dismissive diagnosis of testosterone-loss in older men is 'depression', the modern default for medical 'I don't know'.

In many cases, depression is indeed present but the idea that low testosterone and its symptoms might be the cause is very rarely considered.

Testosterone-Poverty victims are thus condemned to live frustrated, confused and anguished lives simply because those who should most help them are ignorant of their condition and treating them the wrong way.

One GP I asked also suggested that many practitioners are loathe to interact with male genitals even though loss of libido is a very clear indication of Testosterone-Poverty and thus should be a clear pointer to deeper investigation of a man's hormone levels.

Only if a man is brave enough to ask for help with erectile dysfunction will he be likely to be offered testosterone replacement and then only if he has attended a specialist clinic, because his GP 'doesn't feel qualified'.

Think, then, what any sensitive and already embarrassed man feels when he discovers he must sit in a public-hospital waiting-room beneath a large sign saying: Erectile Dysfunction Clinic. This happened to me at a major London hospital very recently, even though I had never complained about this problem. When I queried why I was there rather than at the main Endocrinology Clinic I was told this was because sexual malfunction was the most common problem with older men with testosterone issues. Yet again, decisions were being made about me with no discussion and thus with no empathetic understanding of reality.

Erectile dysfunction wasn't my prime problem. I wanted reassurance that the level of Testosterone-Replacement Therapy I was prescribed would maintain my mind's competence. Being mentally competent is much more important to me than hoping to reproduce teenage virility. I want to continue to be me, to be a writer, for as long as I can.

Overall, I found men with testosterone loss were less concerned about sex and more about their ability to do what might be called more public 'men' things, such as their ability to drive, to be financially competent and not to be bad-tempered, risking the comfort of long-term relationships at the time they needed them most.

Mental Turmoil, Physical Torture

Knowledge about testosterone seems not to have improved in the first two decades of the 21st century. Every GP to whom I have spoken about Testosterone-Poverty has asked for copies of this book, admitting the effects of this state are little known to them. There is constant proof this is so.

In 2018 in Sydney, Australia, a friend in his mid-70s was discovered to have diminished bone-density/osteoporosis. When a man's testosterone is removed as routine treatment for prostate cancer, it's common to test for this condition; it's one of the few widely recognised symptoms of Testosterone-Poverty. Thus it seems obvious that any ageing man with osteoporosis should have his testosterone level checked, in case this is a contributing factor. Yet, when my friend asked for his testosterone levels to be measured, his female GP asked: What's the point?

She dismissed further discussion, almost certainly in my opinion because she feared questions about virility and male genitalia. Even GPs don't seem to believe that old people want sex or should be allowed to enjoy sex, perhaps confusing this with every child's horror at the thought of their parents 'doing it'.

They do. So do their grandparents and uncles and aunties.

Such ignorance or disinterest by medics is why today's Silent Hordes suffer the same harrowing and unrelieved mental turmoil, physical torture, social derision and isolation as history's Invisible Hordes of adult-made eunuchs, those castrated men without the testosterone they once had, who served the Greek, Roman, Byzantine, Ottoman and Chinese empires – and most Eastern countries in between, especially in the many dynasties and empires of India.

The father of another friend in Australia has been very ill for the last 10 years and is now bedridden because of his bad reaction to chemical castration and the nasty effects of radiotherapy.

Then as recently as January 2019 I was told about a UK man in his early 80s, who has 'quickly disintegrated from a bright, full-of-life retired, successful business man into a shell of a man empty of confidence, unable to put words together to make sentences and suffering, amongst other things, uncomfortable hot flushes'. That's seems heartlessly cruel treatment of a man that age and is proof of the need for vigilance; testosterone is so unpredictable it's not just younger men who have such extreme reactions to its suppression.

Scared of What is Happening

The 21st-century's burgeoning populace of aged men with testosterone that has naturally reduced to castrate level or close is vast, but their miseries are largely unrecognised even in the most medically advanced countries and that's why I am going to repeat myself, so the message is clear.

The family, friends and colleagues of Age-related Testosterone-Paupers commonly suffer quite as much as each victim, because none is medically sophisticated enough to understand that testosterone loss is behind the changes they see those men experiencing.

Testosterone-Poverty might well be why that wonderful life-partner has not mellowed with age but has become cantankerous, perhaps even angry enough to be belligerent.

Losing testosterone has widely different effects, from relief at no longer having to compete in work or play to anguish at now harbouring a penis that prefers watching a man polish shoes rather than watching him shave.

With lessening testosterone there are fewer drives for the elderly man to win, or, even, to compete. In extremis there can be so little testosterone that accountants find themselves unable to count, golfers unable to golf and builders unable to build, because measurements, calculating distance, understanding money, playing Bridge and driving safely all become challenges rather than careless skills. Bones crumble, dementia and depression threaten and breasts can develop as their body relentlessly feminises.

Men are confused when these changes happen and are commonly accused of being aggressive when they are actually frightened and angry, age-related short-term memory loss doesn't help. The changes to their bodies do not engender easy acceptance but more readily inflame bad temper and over-assertiveness.

These men are scared of what is happening, and it seems there are few GPs who can explain it to them.

The Trans-Gendering Reality

Physically, a man whose attrition of testosterone is profound becomes the equivalent of a post-menopausal woman.

Uncle Bob really does become your Auntie, pink-cheeked and plump-bottomed, with female patterns of fat deposits and feminine smoothness of skin, at very least; his body hair is likely to be finer or to disappear and he certainly won't need to shave his softened beard as often.

Sadly, benign temperament, kindness and sweetness are not always present when this virtual trans-gendering takes place gradually. Imagine how destructive this can be in a long-term gay relationship, when the two men are both suffering but undiagnosed.

It doesn't have to be this way. To change this, today's Silent Horde of Testosterone-Paupers and the women and men in their lives must start shouting.

The need for compassion, for accurate diagnosis and for Testosterone-Replacement Therapy is often greater if a man's Testosterone-Poverty has been artificially created as treatment for prostate cancer.

That's because it's sudden, brutish and never calibrated to the individual or to his age. The younger the man, the greater the awful side effects are likely to be. See: What Testosterone-Poverty Did To Me.

II:Prostate Cancer Testosterone-Paupers

The World Cancer Research Fund says prostate cancer is the second most common cancer in men and the fourth most common cancer overall.

Prostate cancer attacks more than 10% of men in Caucasian populations and very many more in African heritage men. More than 100 men are diagnosed with it every day in the UK, over 500 a day in the United States, so that's over 36,000 every year in the UK, more than 182,000 every year in the USA. In other countries the percentile rate is two to three times higher and that is only those who have been medically diagnosed.

These numbers are just the new cases and every year there are carry-overs of those still being treated and those who are suffering the long-term effects of Testosterone-Poverty after prostate-cancer therapies.

It is not exaggerating to say that at any hour of any day there are millions of men worldwide who are Prostate-Cancer Testosterone-Paupers, four words that reverberate endlessly with misery. It's astonishing that treatment for cancer in such a small human organ can cause so much desolation.

Tunnel Vision to Despair

The adult male's prostate gland, no bigger than a smooth, hard walnut or small apricot if healthy, sits directly on the outside of the final length of the large intestine, between it and the bladder. Internally, it is but a finger-length away.

The prostate's orgasm, which ameliorates the acidity of sperm with milky-sweet fluids, is contemporary with an ejaculating erection's few seconds of intensity and contributes about 20% of the ejaculate volume. There is a double-seated sense of pleasure that seamlessly joins in the entire length of the penis, past the testicles and into its thicker anchor between the legs. Thinking a penis starts and finishes in front of the scrotum is a common misconception, half-cocked you might say.

Much of the medical profession believes that testosterone encourages the growth of prostate cancers and so this critical hormone is commonly demolished before any other treatments for the tumour, no matter how young or old the patient, how small the tumour is or how early it has been identified.

If the connection is true in any degree, this means that silently and with spiteful irony, the very testosterone that created each man may be what hastens him back to dust, just as naturally but infinitely more unpleasantly.

Once a tumour is confirmed, chemical castration is prescribed and is known in clinics and hospitals as Testosterone-Hormone Therapy. This hormone-repressing therapy, which is far from therapeutic for most men, is probably unnecessary in many cases. It is applied in broad swipes, rarely related to the individual patient or calibrated to the state and size of his tumour.

These chemical castrations cause life-changing effects on patients, partners and families that can be catastrophic. The side-effects are widely ignored because of tunnel-vision views that killing the cancer outweighs all other considerations of a patient's social or business welfare.

Evidence Refuted and Dismissed

It is reasonable to suggest that hormone-removal 'therapy' is often prescribed by oncologists as a form of self-protection, a selfish guard for their reputation at the expense of the well-being of their patients, regardless of those men's intellectual ability or if there are support systems in place to help them.

This broadly based use of testosterone suppression is increasingly condemned because of growing concerns that testosterone has little to do with the genesis of prostate cancer, largely because what evidence there is for the connection is over half a century old. The oncologist presumably fears being accused of bad practice if the tumour should suddenly erupt between diagnosis and the delay common before treatment with radiotherapy or chemotherapy. So, the patient is sacrificed, as I certainly felt, with no advice on or knowledge of what might happen or for how long when their testosterone is abolished. And absolutely no guidance on when or if it will return.

Prostate-Cancer Testosterone-Paupers and their futures can be particularly wretched and yet, in spite of their enormous numbers, most are untreated for the side-effects of testosterone removal.

Often, as happened to me, the obvious physical and mental effects might not even be accepted as associated with testosterone suppression, a stance supported for a long time by drug manufacturers, who refuted overwhelming contrary evidence, especially relating to therapy-caused depression. You will today find grudging advice on both drug packaging and in hospital literature, suggesting that 'mood changes' might be a symptom of testosterone suppression. This is far from being a 'proper' warning.

Many millions are spent on research into new ways to detect and to treat prostate-cancer, largely because the effects of radiotherapy's permanent scarring of the bladder and bowels can be severe, life changing and life-long. Yet, little seems to be done about the short and long-term effects of Testosterone-Hormone Therapy.

Forgive more repetition but it's vital never to forget that irresponsible testosterone suppression destroys relationships and marriages, because penetrative, penis-led sex is vanquished, spatial skills are attenuated, careers are suddenly ended, sports prowess nullified.

Such men are modern victims of a type of castration that has as little subtlety as a castrator's tools, and they are unrecognised as 21st-century eunuchs. Every untreated contemporary eunuch, created chemically or naturally by ageing, or through accident or disease, becomes as unreliable or inadequate as any engine without fuel, whether inherently moped or Maserati.

It shouldn't be like this, particularly not if testosterone replacement, HRT for MEN is given soon after treatment for the tumour, something oncologists are wary about doing. This is particularly wicked because the research that accepts that testosterone promotes the growth of prostate cancer is now highly suspected as being either wrong or over-emphasised. Money and minds would be better spent using modern forensic research to determine the truth. At very least, methods should be developed to calibrate testosterone suppression, according to the size of the tumour and perhaps even to the size and age of the man, a widely held view among patients and others to whom I spoke, including those working in prostate-cancer charities.

Tumour Death is Not Enough

Testosterone suppression means a man who is already struggling with his awful diagnosis of cancer and how this is affecting his life is thoughtlessly also expected to battle the effects of the 'therapy', from loss of libido to hot flashes, mental incapacities and degrees of mood change and depression that can mean loss of employment and thus of being unable to support dependants.

If he undergoes radiotherapy he will almost certainly also suffer both bladder and bowel incontinence. Without exception these are the side effects that men most dread and that most drain them of whatever remaining feelings they have of masculinity or maturity. Radiotherapy incontinence, caused by burning of tissue by the treatment, is likely to be permanent and can make a man very unhappy, particularly when it inhibits his social life. Isolation can become very appealing, even though based on shame and self-loathing. It's further diminishing to find that pharmacies, even big branches of Boots or Superdrug, often have many shelves of incontinence pads for women but not a single product for men. This vastly underpins the feeling that the lesser-man you find yourself to be is not worth bothering about by the rest of the world, neither medically nor socially.

Enduring incontinence is an inescapable price that prostate-cancer victims must accept, in return for being cured, for being alive. That makes it even more important that the equally diminishing effects of Testosterone-Poverty should be addressed and solved, truly giving a degree of Quality of Life to a patient, rather than settling into complacent self-congratulation simply because the tumour has been defeated.

The death of the tumour is NOT enough.

The Difficulty of Complaint

Young or old, it requires an unusually determined man to complain and question his doctor about testosterone-related symptoms when otherwise seeming to be well. It's even harder for a man who has been told he is alive only because of the prostate-cancer treatments he has undergone.

While I was being treated, I saw that it was working-class men, those with the least likelihood of financial security, medical sophistication or communicative skills, who were the least likely to ask for relief from the symptoms of testosterone loss, probably not wishing to admit weakness, that they were not feeling the man they once were.

Anecdotally, in London anyway, black men seemed even more likely to suffer, partly because of a cultural machoism of men not complaining, particularly about anything to do with their genitals; young black men with older relatives who were prostate-cancer victims despaired of the private pain endured because their older family members, male and female, were not able to complain or even to put their agony into words in front of a doctor. In all cases, the effects on their family life were likely to be even more horrid than the expected upheaval during treatment.

Fairer, Kinder, Better

If the effort and money that goes into breast-cancer research and treatment were to be balanced by similar research into the truth about the true effect of testosterone on prostate cancer, the result could show that Testosterone-Replacement Therapy should be used as soon as treatments are over, restoring a man's identity and his place in his family and in the world.

That would make a fairer, kinder and better world for modern men.

And for women and children, too.

International Incidence of Prostate Cancer, 2018

Published by The World Cancer Research Fund, this chart gives the barest indication of the number of men who will suffer the enervating, sometimes permanent ill-effects both of radiology or chemotherapy as well as of the loss of their essential male hormone.

Rank	Country	Age-standardised rate per 1,000
1	Guadeloupe (France)	189.1
2	Martihique (France)	158.4
3	Ireland	132.5
4	Barbados	129.3
5	Estonia	109.9
6	Norway	106.5
7	Sweden	103.0
8	Puerto Rico	101.7
9	France (metropolitan)	99.0
10	New Calidonia (France)	93.0

Rank	Country	Age-standardised rate per 1,000
11	French Guiana	92.3
12	New Zealand	90.8
13	Czech Republic	88.0
14	Bahamas	85.8
15	Australia	85.6
16	United Kingdom	80.7
17	Latvia	80.3
18	Slovenia	79.3
19	Luxembourg	78.8
20	Switzerland	77.4

Source: Bray F, Ferlay J, Soerjomataram I, Siegel RL, Torre LA, Jemal A. Global Cancer Statistics 2018: GLOBOCAN estimates of incidence and mortality worldwide for 36 cancers in 185 countries. CA Cancer J Clin, in press. The online GLOBOCAN 2018 database is accessible at http://gco. larc.fr/ as part of IARC's Global Cancer Observatory.

III: Chemical Testosterone-Paupers

These are created when testosterone-stifling chemicals are pre-scribed to neuter sex criminals or to support trans-gendering from male to female.

These latter ex-males have their symptoms alleviated by the administration of female hormones and generally suffer least from testosterone loss.

IV: Trauma Testosterone-Paupers

Young and old, these are men whose testicles have been de-stroyed by trauma, perhaps in a car crash or through an accident on a bicycle, horse, skate-board or sporting incident.

The mental struggle they have to accept their new state can be enormous, as it can for the next categories.

V: Hero Testosterone-Paupers

These victims are those serving soldiers whose testicles have been cruelly injured or ripped from them by enemy action, perhaps the least acknowledged of all modern castrates.

It's hoped these returning young heroes would be particularly likely to have testosterone-replacement therapy, but apocryphal stories from serving men make this seem not always to be the case.

VI: Disease or Disorder-Related Testosterone-Paupers

Diseases or disorders that cause absolute Testosterone-Poverty or Hypo-gonadism are divided into two. Primary Hypo-gonadism is when the condition is caused by a malfunction of the testicles. Disease or Disorder-related Testosterone-Paupers include men who have suffered testicular cancer and had their testicles surgically removed, a procedure called orchiectomy.

If the problem is based in the pituitary gland it is known as Secondary Hypo-gonadism. Pituitary-gland issues, including tumours, can cause Testosterone-Poverty because this gland controls the manufacture of testosterone in the testicles, a process easily obliterated.

Younger men classically develop low testosterone levels through Type 2 diabetes, chronic liver or kidney diseases, and COPD or other lung disease.

Today we must add HIV infections and the stupidity of steroid overuse; it's common to find that men with the biggest muscles based on steroid intake commonly have the least libido or sexual performance because the drugs have destroyed their ability to manufacture testosterone.

Unfortunate genetic disorders include Klinefelter syndrome, Kallmann syndrome, Prader-Willi syndrome and Myotonic syndrome. With few exceptions these low-testosterone conditions are recognised and treatable but that's only because their other symptoms have first been acknowledged.

The Emperor's Breasts
Historically and today, Disease or Disorder-related Testosterone-Poverty can assault a man at any age. Even if he is a war hero and has declared himself an emperor, a man without testosterone

will feminise. When Napoleon Bonaparte died in 1821 on St Helena he was 51. It is well documented that his genitals had shrunk and that his breasts were considered more beautiful than those of either of his empresses, but who said this proved impossible to find.

Once renowned as an ardent love maker, Bonaparte said himself that his interest rather withered after his second marriage in 1810 to Marie-Louise, a Hapsburg princess, although he did father a son and putative heir born in 1811, when he was about 41. Called the King of Rome at birth, and expected to become Napoleon II, the son died in exile as the Duke of Reichstadt in 1832.

One of the doctors who examined the emperor's body supposedly said: 'His type of plumpness was not masculine; he had beautiful arms, rounded breasts, white soft skin (and) no hair.' Other writers point out that he always had the typical feminine shape of narrow shoulders and wide hips and this can be seen in innumerable portraits, even when his body is disguised by uniforms and sumptuous robes of golden imperial splendour. His later, further plumped buttocks and emboldened breasts meant that he once was mistaken for the elderly governess of his second wife, the Empress Marie-Louise.

One explanation of Bonaparte's problem might be a long-term pituitary-gland disorder, because this gland controls the manufacture of testosterone in the testicles. If true, his condition was an extreme Disease or Disorder-related case of what otherwise happens naturally but more slowly to ageing men as their testosterone levels drop.

A 21st-century Tale of Testosterone-Poverty

It's hard to think the following story is true, yet I believe it. Clearly the man's first replacement doses were too high and are now too low. Compare that to the enormous industry supporting hormone replacement for women – and wonder.

From: *The Guardian* April 13, 2018

"I was diagnosed with testicular cancer 23 years ago, when I was 31, and both balls were removed. I had been in a relationship for six months, but it ended soon after and there's been no one since. I was treated with a hormone-replacement therapy which caused relentless erections; lonely and horny is a miserable combination. I started watching pornography because it was safe and there was no fear of humiliation, but it only reinforced my sense of isolation.

"The treatment was withdrawn because of its side-effects – obesity, aggression, sexual rampancy – and since being put on a "safer" type of testosterone, I've been impotent. I began visiting escort girls for a kiss and a cuddle, lying with them in my arms. I'd call a chatline and have fake phone sex, pretending to orgasm at the appropriate point in the charade. I've fantasised about fantasies, acted out roles of virile masculinity, wretchedly impersonated a man. Recently I began making politely inept passes at gorgeous girls, emboldened by inevitable dismissal; another sham pantomime.

"I have nothing else to declare – I'm a sexual nonentity. I began counselling in January and wish I had been referred 20 years ago. The anguish never stops, so I've learned to repress dangerous emotions. I admire women abstractly but occasionally one slips through my defences and destroys me; I'll find her incredibly attractive, want her desperately, but have no outlet for the powerful feelings that surge up within me. I weep uncontrollably when I imagine being with her, sweet desire unleashing all the shame, rage and despair inside me."

PART VI

The HRT for MEN Imperatives

More Than Recommendations

The only way that Quality of Life will improve for Testosterone-Paupers is to get the subject out into the air, to talk about it, shout about it.

Get that done and we are on the way to alleviating untold despair, heartbreak and potential suicides.

The extra years that men now live should have as much quality about them as all the others or what is the point of being alive?

Following are recommendations for what women, men, GPs, oncologists, andrologists and endocrinologists should do to make this a reality.

More than recommendations, the following three lists must be imperatives if 55+ Men's Health and that of their families and colleagues are all to be released from any unnecessary bondage of Testosterone-Poverty.

Testosterone-Replacement Therapy is life changing, lifesaving, just as Hormone-Replacement Therapy, HRT, is for millions of women, who now gratefully lead fuller and more fulfilled lives because of it.

Where are the raging millions of men demanding HRT/TRT as their right? Or the women making them demand it?

I: HRT Imperatives
For Women

- Check the men in your life from 55-years old for signs of Testosterone-Poverty: learn these from my Catechism of Testosterone-Poverty

- Tell the men in your life who are 55+ or more to ask for testosterone-level checks at least once a year, ideally at the same time as the PSA blood test, which detects possible prostate cancer

- Tell your GP that you would like testosterone levels checked in your husband, father, grandfather, boyfriend, partner, grandson, nephew, son, son or daughter's boyfriend, any of them if they are 55+

- Ensure prostate-cancer patients have their testosterone levels recorded before treatment.

- Don't believe everything that a drug company says: question, question, question

- Resist automatic testosterone-suppression before prostate-cancer therapy until a second opinion says it is truly needed and even so support the man if he continues not to want this

- Demand Testosterone-Replacement Therapy as soon as possible after prostate-cancer treatment if testosterone has been removed

- Do not be afraid to remind oncologists that recurrence of the cancer after testosterone-suppression is rare and that regular blood tests would show this if it does happen – in the meantime the Quality of Life of your 55+ man and all around him will be immeasurably improved

- Read and remember everything in HRT Imperatives for Men

- Tell other women about Testosterone-Poverty in 55+ men

II: HRT Imperatives For Men

- After 55+, be aware of physical and mental failings as listed in my Catechism of Testosterone-Poverty

- Don't be a wimp. Tell your doctor of any suspicions. Ask directly for a blood test to check for low testosterone levels

- Insist on having your testosterone levels checked annually, ideally when having your annual or bi-annual PSA test for prostate cancer

- Ensure your testosterone level is recorded before any treatment for prostate cancer

- Don't believe everything a drug company says about side effects; question, question, question

- Resist automatic testosterone-suppression before prostate-cancer therapy until a second opinion says it is truly needed and even so insist on not having this treatment if that is your wish

- Demand Testosterone-Replacement Therapy as soon after possible after treatment for prostate cancer that includes hormone (testosterone) removal

- Do not be afraid to remind oncologists that recurrence of the cancer because of Testosterone-Replacement Therapy after testosterone-suppression is rare and that regular blood tests would show this if it does happen – in the meantime your Quality of Life and that of those around you will be immeasurably improved

- Tell family, friends, colleagues and neighbours about Testosterone-Poverty, especially 55+ men.

III: HRT Imperatives for Doctors, Oncologists, Andrologists and Endrocronologists

- Keep up-to-date with modern thinking about testosterone and testosterone replacement therapies

- Test all 55+ male patients annually for lowered testosterone levels, ideally when also PSA testing

- Prescribe Testosterone-Replacement Therapy to 55+ patients with low levels of testosterone and then monitor

- Actively consider Testosterone-Poverty as a likely cause of many symptoms in 55+ ageing men, especially of lowered mood or depression; see my Catechism of Testosterone-Poverty Symptoms

- Record testosterone levels before prostate-cancer treatments

- Resist automatic testosterone-suppression before prostate-cancer therapy until a second opinion says it is truly necessary but still allow a patient to refuse if they wish

- Prescribe Testosterone-Replacement Therapy to prostate-cancer patients soon after their surgical, radiotherapy or chemotherapy treatments are completed, especially younger ones of 55 to 65.

- Then use blood tests regularly to monitor testosterone and PSA levels

- Remember that recurrence of prostate cancer because of Testosterone-Replacement Therapy after testosterone suppression is rare and that regular blood tests would show this if it does happen – in the meantime your patients' Quality of Life will be immeasurably improved

- Quality of Life should be just as much a target as death of a tumour

- Tell your colleagues, professional and governing bodies about Testosterone-Replacement Therapies

- Don't believe everything a drug company tells you; question, question, question.

Caution

This is not an academic paper or a medical casebook but a summary of my experiences, observations and thought. Testosterone-Replacement Therapy will indeed solve many of the mental and physical problems of 55+ men, reduce the side effects of hormone therapy in prostate-cancer patients and help restore vitality and a sense of normality in every aspect of daily life to Testosterone-Paupers.

Yet, Testosterone-Poverty is not the only cause of the many symptoms and complaints that come with 55+ Men's Health, including depression or erectile dysfunction.

The critical message of this book is that identifying Testosterone-Poverty must become a normal tool in the path to diagnosis of 55+ Men's Health.

A simple blood test will at once establish the facts and should be insisted on, by every 55+ man, by the men and women who love him and, most of all, by his medical professionals.

Testosterone-Replacement Therapy should then become as commonplace for men as HRT is for women.

That would be an important step forward in the 21st-century's continuing journey towards equal value and Quality of Life everywhere for its men and women.

Glynn Christian
www.glynnchristian.com

Glynn Christian was a pioneering BBC-TV chef (Pebble Mill, BBC Breakfast Time *et al)* and helped found the UK Guild of Food Writers.

REAL FLAVOURS – *The Handbook of Gourmet and Deli Ingredients* (Grub Street) was voted World's Best Food Guide at Le Cordon Bleu World Food Media Awards. Nigel Slater called it 'one of the only ten books you need': Tom Parker Bowles says it is 'as important to the kitchen as a sharp knife'. Glynn was subsequently honoured with a Lifetime Achievement Award by the Guild of Fine Foods, the only food writer given such an honour. His latest food-based book is HOW TO COOK WITHOUT RECIPES (Portico).

He is a gt gt gt gt grandson of Fletcher Christian, leader of the 1789 mutiny on HMAV BOUNTY and of Mauatua, his Tahitian consort.

FRAGILE PARADISE - *The Discovery of Fletcher Christian,* BOUNTY *Mutineer* (1982, 1999 and 2007) is the only biography of his ancestor among over 3500 books and major articles about the world's best-known mutiny and it has become seminal reference for any author writing about BOUNTY.

MRS CHRISTIAN – BOUNTY MUTINEER is his first historical-fiction book: Mauatua Christian directed bloody revolution on Pitcairn Island and in 1838 led the island's women to be first in the world to vote and to make education compulsory for girls. A collage-opera (*pasticcio*) about Mrs Christian is being worked on, using only late-18th century English baroque music (mainly Handel) and Tahitian rhythms and harmonies of the time.

He now lives in London where until recently he was a volunteer guide at the Victoria and Albert Museum and is currently finishing a book called VICTORIA'S NOBLE NEIGHBOURS, 1885 – *Where London's Lords and Ladies Lived at the Height of Imperial Splendour.*

CREDITS

Cover and book design: Andrew Smith, who was also a completely reliable editor and is the very best of mates.

Grateful thanks for encouragement, criticisms and corrections to: Anne Dolamore, Bob Farrand, Michael Binyon, Matthew Nowell, Daniel Nowell, Merville Spiers, Sue Christian, Faye Christian, Kerry Bevin and dear Camilla Osborne